The Dementia Handbook

The Dementia Handbook

HOW TO PROVIDE DEMENTIA CARE AT HOME

Judy Cornish

Dementia & Alzheimer's Wellbeing Network® (DAWN)

ISBN: 1541326555
ISBN 13: 9781541326552
Library of Congress Control Number: 2016921439
CreateSpace Independent Publishing Platform
North Charleston, South Carolina

Debby Dodds, MS
Gerontologist
Dementia is an epidemic and a care challenge. This book helps us re-frame the dementia dialog. As Judy so eloquently points out, "Loved ones don't stop experiencing things just because they cannot recall or recount them." When caregivers respectfully focus on current abilities and provide choice, the results are rewarding. As a gerontologist and as a daughter, I have been using Judy's DAWN Method successfully for over a year. I hope that you, too, will find success in this approach.

Glenda Hawley, MSW, PhD
Psychotherapist & Grief Counselor
I have watched Judy Cornish work with several clients in our community, both as a friend and professional, and have seen the effectiveness of her innovative approach to dementia care. I have seen the well-being her clients exhibit as well as the peace and confidence families gain in learning how to approach their loved one with understanding. As a professional, I am looking forward to using this book as a reference and recommending it to appropriate clients.

Patricia Sublette, PhD
Special Education & Traumatic Brain Injury Specialist
This book equips families to provide excellent dementia care at home. Judy Cornish's approach integrates knowledge from diverse fields to help families provide targeted support for loved ones losing executive functioning and memory. Her DAWN Method creates a respectful, personalized approach that honors each individual who experiences Alzheimer's or dementia.

This book is dedicated to my clients, who courageously face dementia every day and honor me with the task of helping them preserve happiness and dignity.

The power of intuitive understanding will
protect you from harm until
the end of your days.

Lao Tzu

Contents

CHAPTER 1

Bad, but Not All Bad

I n the past six years, I've spent more time with people who have dementia than with people who don't. I'm writing this book to explain what they taught me.

I feel more like a scribe than an author in writing it. Of course, we can only learn what our brains are equipped to understand. What we already believe to be true influences how we interpret new information. Up to six years ago, my experiences and education did not include dementia care. They included practicing law, working a few years with the mentally ill and brain injured, and studying literature, languages, and art. What I saw and heard from my dementia clients was not preceded by a degree in medicine or social work. So, at the end of this book, you will find a list of the authors and books that shaped how I interpreted what my clients with dementia came to teach me. Here, at the beginning, I will summarize why I think it's so important for us to listen to what the people who have dementia are telling us and why we need to do a better job helping them.

Dementia Is an Epidemic

Zika, Ebola, and HIV have gotten more press, but too many people in the United States are developing dementia for us to ignore this condition of progressive cognitive impairment. In 2015, the estimate was 5.3 million people. This means that at least 5.3 million families were trying to live with someone who was failing at daily life with increasing regularity, with no hope of improvement. We haven't yet reached the height of the epidemic. Right now, someone is diagnosed with dementia about every sixty-six seconds. By 2030, the estimate is every thirty-three seconds.

Because dementia is progressive and incurable, eventually families find they cannot keep their loved ones safe at home and must put them into institutional care. Paying for care at home is expensive, but the cost of long-term care in facilities is astronomical.

Institutional Care Is Expensive

The average cost of a shared room in a memory care facility in 2015 was $90,500. Most of us can't cover an expense like that indefinitely. In 2012, American families spent over $49 billion on long-term services and supports. Medicare spends about three times more on beneficiaries who have dementia than on those who don't. The most recent estimate I could find in terms of dollars was for 2013: the bill to Medicare was $107 billion for health care for dementia patients.

When families run out of money to pay for long-term care, state Medicaid programs step in. During 2012, Medicaid programs paid about $134 billion for long-term care services and support, which was about 31 percent of all Medicaid spending.

With an estimated 70 percent of people aged sixty-five and older needing long-term care—and people aged over eighty-five being our fastest-growing population segment—we have a problem. Quite simply, most of us will need long-term care, but few of us can afford it. The reality is that many of us will be forced to stay home, with our families doing the best they can to care for our needs.

We need to be equipped to provide dementia care safely and economically. The good news is that there is an approach that makes it easier to live with dementia, without institutional care.

We Can Learn to Live with It

There is a very real stigma to admitting that you are becoming cognitively impaired. If people know you have a diagnosis of Alzheimer's or dementia, they look at you oddly, wondering if you'll do or say something bizarre. If they don't know your diagnosis, they can't help but notice when you begin to repeat yourself or make comments that are out of place in conversation. They see your mistakes as you attempt to navigate daily life without memory. Among my friends and the families I have worked with, diagnosis is usually put off and then not acknowledged until after the person has learned to isolate and avoid new situations in order to escape embarrassment.

In responding to dementia with avoidance and denial, we unwittingly exacerbate our loved ones' predicament. If we try to pretend they are functioning as usual, their failures and growing disabilities are glaringly exposed. On the other hand, if we were to embrace the presence of dementia as bringing a specific set of disabilities, we could focus on helping our loved ones and clients develop the skills and abilities they have left. When people lose eyesight, we don't avoid the topic of blindness and wait for their self-care to deteriorate; we help them navigate without sight and learn to read with their fingers. When people lose hearing, we don't expect them to hear as best they can; we alter their environment so that they can still be safe and help them learn to read lips. So, when someone loses memory and rational thought, why don't we take care of those functions for them and help them become better at using the intuitive skills that remain?

We Can Live with It, Because Not Everything Is Lost

I have never heard from a client or family dealing with dementia that a medical professional, social worker, or senior-care specialist told them there was good news about dementia. I have had a number of families tell me that I was the first person to offer them hope or a road map to follow as they sought to guide their loved ones through the cognitive changes that would come. I think there is good news regarding dementia, although it's not actually new; it's just not widely acknowledged in the United States.

The old but good news is *habilitative care*. We say we are using habilitative care when we approach caring for people experiencing dementia by evaluating their personal limitations and their perception of reality, and then changing their environment to make it more supportive of their emotional needs and cognitive abilities. Habilitative care has been written about since the early 1990s. It's widely in use in Commonwealth countries and Europe. In using it, caregivers accept that loss of memory and rational thought alters their charges' ability to perceive reality.

The default manner of providing dementia care in the United States has been an approach referred to as *appropriate care* and *reality orientation*, which means that people with dementia are corrected if their belief about what is real or happening differs from reality. Caregivers using the habilitative dementia care approach do not do this. Rather than ask people to function in a normal environment and accept reality as if they had healthy brains, habilitative caregivers pay attention to the individual's specific and changing needs—altering the physical environment as necessary and accepting the skewed perception of reality that progressive cognitive impairment causes. This is true dementia care, care that works with both the disabilities and the abilities of dementia. Because this care provides an individualized response to each person's specific and changing needs, we refer to it as *person-directed care.*

The good but unacknowledged news is that although memory and rational thought begin to melt away early in dementia, the intuitive thought processes do not. Further, our intuitive thought processes include some of the most enjoyable ones we have: the ability to recognize our own feelings and those of others, the ability to enjoy music and creativity, and the ability to perceive and enjoy beauty. Our fight-or-flight reactions also remain, something caregivers are wise to remember when working with people whose rational thought is fading away.

We don't know how long a person's intuitive thought processes remain. I don't think we've conducted studies to explore the question yet, as with much else in the world of dementia care. It would be prudent, then, to assume that intuitive thought remains until death, because that would lead caregivers to treat people with respect and compassion even when they become bedridden and unable to communicate. Think of how much pain and indignity people may be suffering in the final stages of dementia because their caregivers do not consider whether they are still experiencing the present.

So, I propose that we see dementia as a devastating condition, one that causes great expense to families, Medicare, and Medicaid, but not a hopeless one. If we provide habilitative care and educate ourselves about the skills and abilities that people with dementia retain, we can maximize function, preserve dignity, and keep our loved ones at home longer. We can make their lives (and ours) much better than we're doing at present.

In law school, I learned to look at what appears to be random and unresolvable as an indication that I should search for deeper, unifying factors. In other words, I looked for a pattern. I learned another principle when studying language—that our brains respond in orderly ways and that our errors are logical results of what we have previously learned or experienced. In the same way, I believe we should expect dementia-related behaviors to be logical and predictable expressions of the individual's emotional needs. If we identify what lies beneath, a pattern emerges, and disorder dissolves into predictability.

Let's now look at those skills and abilities that are lost in dementia and those that remain. We will find a pattern that makes dementia care less stressful.

CHAPTER 2

Not All Is Lost

Dementia is defined as cognitive impairment that may result from injury or several diseases, is ongoing, and eventually interferes with daily life to the point that full care is necessary. This is accurate but not helpful for those of us who are trying to live with someone experiencing dementia. We need to know which functions will stay and which will go, in practical terms. Being able to live and work happily with people who have dementia requires knowing when to help and how. There are some functions that everyone loses to dementia. Which, exactly, are those?

What Is Lost?

Memory

Usually memory goes first. In working with my clients, I've come to think of memory loss in three broad groups: memories that disappear, memories that become altered, and false memories that are essentially some form of déjà vu (the feeling that something has happened before). This last category seems to be a stage that lasts a few months and then doesn't reappear, so it doesn't have the impact the other two memory problems present.

It is lost memories and altered memories that wreak havoc in relationships and daily routines, because they dramatically change the person's belief of what is true in the present—in other words, the perception of reality. This creates an immediate and constant friction between caregiver and care receiver.

If a husband has lost the memory of having agreed at breakfast time to fill the car with gas and have it packed and ready to leave for the weekend when his wife gets home, both parties will be upset. She will be upset not only because he's failed to do what he agreed to do but also because he has behaved in a way inconsistent with her expectations formed over many years of marriage. If he does not believe he has memory problems, he will feel unjustly accused and be upset that she has expectations that are not based on reality. (People with dementia may also have *anosognosia*, the condition of being unaware and unable to perceive that they have impairments.) Both will be able to honestly search their memories and come up with a recollection that feels accurate, but one will recall the conversation, and the other will recall the absence of the conversation.

So, both will feel justifiably indignant. And if the husband is aware of his memory loss, they'll both feel fear at this indication of his growing impairment. Memories that either fail to get recorded in the first place or become inaccessible later start appearing early in dementia.

Further into dementia, memories will be randomly altered with no warning or predictability. That same husband may wake up one morning believing that he has always walked downtown for coffee rather than driven. Maybe this mistaken recollection originated in a dream; maybe it came from an early-life memory; maybe it is the result of a random neuron misfiring deep in his brain. In any case, he will now search his memory and find that feeling of surety that accompanies the knowledge that he has done something many times before. Trying to convince him otherwise isn't likely to work. Both husband and wife will experience keen annoyance due to their differing versions of reality when she tries to convince him that such a walk would be dangerous and exhausting.

When what we believe to be true differs from what those around us believe, it is upsetting for both us and them. Changes in memory begin early in dementia, and the most devastating casualty is losing the ability to stay grounded in common reality.

The Remembering Self

We don't think of ourselves as having a remembering self and an experiential self, but if we are living or working with people who have dementia, we need to start.

Think about various people you know and how they choose vacations and leisure activities. Some people seek experiences. They are always looking for something new and exciting. Others like to repeat past vacations that were enjoyable and rich in pleasant memories. The former group heads off to a different exotic destination each year, while the latter returns to the same beach cottage summer after summer. The first might forget to take pictures while away, yet the second finds as much enjoyment in the photo album as on the beach.

This happens because we all have an experiential self as well as a remembering self. The experiential self is the part of us that is in the moment having experiences. The remembering self is the part of us that can look back and recall what went before. We each have a preference for one or the other, but we all lose the remembering self when dementia strikes. As caregivers, we err if we assume that the loss of the remembering self means the loss of the experiential self. Dementia takes away the ability to remember, but it does not take away the ability to experience.

Rational Thought Processes

I provide dementia care in a university town in northern Idaho. Whether my clients were professors, artists, housewives, ranchers, or scientists in their earlier years, I have seen them all lose their rational thought processes and retain their intuitive ones. It doesn't seem to matter which they previously preferred or were better at using.

We all start out with both types of thought. Intuitive thought is involuntary, while using rational thought requires a conscious choice. As with our remembering and experiential selves, we all prefer one over the other. A decade or so ago, a quote became popular and was mistakenly attributed to Einstein: "The intuitive mind is a sacred gift and the rational mind is a faithful servant. We have created a society that honors the servant and has forgotten the gift."

I see truth in this quote. We do prize rational thought over intuitive thought. Just think about how much more we respect and economically reward lawyers and surgeons than artists and housewives. My own education spans both art and law. To me, using intuitive thought is like having an array of paints, brushes, and canvases, whereas using rational thought is like having ruled paper and a well-sharpened pencil. I prefer the former but see value in both, for they enable us to complete very different tasks (the first supports discovery while the second achieves goals). Like me, some of my clients preferred using their intuitive thought skills, but all my clients experience distress as they progressively lose rational thought.

Our rational thought skills include such mental abilities as analyzing and organizing information, recognizing similarities and differences in both objects and concepts, and drawing conclusions. Medical science tells us that people with dementia lose such things as judgment, perception, and executive functions, but that doesn't help me very much when I struggle to deal with the man determined to buy new cookware to replace what he's melted on the stove or the woman who doesn't see anything wrong with using her bare hands to scoop poop from the litter box. I need to understand how these losses translate into behavior.

In functional terms, here are the top three rational thought skills my clients begin to have trouble with and eventually completely fail at as their dementia progresses:

Cause and effect

We learn about cause and effect at a very young age. Infants learn from experience what sounds make their parents smile or come at a run. Children learn through experimentation what happens when they fall off bicycles or throw snowballs at older boys. We spend our lives learning from the feedback we get at every turn. And then, when dementia strikes, that feedback stops having meaning.

My client who kept forgetting he had turned the stove on and melted pots couldn't comprehend why I thought a house fire was likely. Another client didn't see why gloves and a coat were necessary on a snowy Tuesday morning in northern Idaho. Both thought

I was being difficult. No amount of explanation regarding cause and effect would give them back the ability to perceive connections between actions and results. I had to find another way to ensure their safety.

Steps in a process, or sequences

When one client suddenly became incontinent, we had to replace her panties with pull-up Depends (the tape-closure ones leaked, and wet pants upset her). However, now when she hurried to the toilet, she found herself sitting there with dry pants and wet Depends. She could not bring to mind the necessary steps to end up back in a pair of dry Depends with her pants up, so she solved the problem creatively.

She waddled into the spare room with her pants and wet Depends around her knees, found her sewing scissors and cut off the Depends, and then pulled her dry pants back up. Being also unable to see cause and effect (that no Depends would soon result in wet pants), she thought her problem was solved. We marveled at her ingenuity and removed her sewing scissors, only to have her waddle into the kitchen and use a butcher knife the next time.

This is how someone who cannot use rational thought will solve problems—creatively, but with no ability to follow steps or evaluate the consequences.

Prioritization

Being able to prioritize needs, tasks, items, or ideas is also a lost skill for my clients. This becomes apparent when we have a deadline, such as getting to an appointment on time or even just getting the trash out before the garbage truck arrives. My client cannot join me in deciding which tasks we must skip to ensure we can meet the deadline. To my client, every action is of equal importance, so my prompting to forego one activity for another seems bossy.

With our healthy brains, we prioritize all the time—ranking each action or idea according to our goals. My clients, however, see no more importance in putting on shoes than in finding a missing earring before leaving the house. They cannot understand why gathering the rotting pears on the ground in the backyard can be postponed while leaving immediately for a distant medical appointment is essential.

My clients' responses are reasonable and predictable given that they cannot perceive cause and effect, visualize sequences, or prioritize ideas and needs. As their caregiver, it's my responsibility not only to use my own rational thought on their behalf but also to use my awareness of their disabilities to accomplish tasks and preserve safety via other means.

Language Skills

Using language means using words and symbols to communicate our ideas to others, whether verbally or in writing. Dementia eventually takes away the ability to use words or symbols. At what point and which language skills go first depends on the disease or injury that caused the dementia, among other factors. Usually caregivers first notice difficulties with word finding. Then, there will be problems such as word substitutions, shrinking vocabulary, grammatical irregularities, and ultimately loss of the ability to comprehend other people's speech.

The way someone with dementia misuses language can look nonsensical, but I believe there is always a pattern that causes the irregular word choice. It's our job to decipher it. A client reported to me that one night at dinner, her loved one said, "I want some paper," while looking at the bowl of mashed potatoes. She responded by offering the potatoes and received a gratified smile. The words "paper" and "potatoes" aren't as unrelated as you might first think: they both begin with "p," have a long "a" sound, and refer to something white. That's a strong pattern.

As caregivers, we should expect creative and unexpected uses of language and strive to understand the meaning behind the word choices. Your loved one is trying to communicate with you, to share with you. It is not "the dementia talking," as one family I worked with insisted.

As dementia caregivers, we need to think creatively. We need to look for the emotion behind our loved ones' words. The need to communicate continues. The message is there, camouflaged behind unexpected language. When we do this, we are using our intuitive skills, not just our rational ones.

Motor Skills

Be careful to watch for the loss of coordination. It can occur suddenly, quite randomly; it may appear permanently or intermittently.

Most of our clients exhibit increased confusion when they get a urinary tract infection (a common problem as people age). For one client, her increased confusion primarily affected her ability to coordinate major muscle groups. If she wanted to get off the toilet, for instance, she might find herself unable to tense her thigh muscles and pull on the handrail at the same time. Worse yet, when she realized she was trapped and called out for help, she couldn't coordinate her arms and legs to help us lift her up and thought we were refusing to help.

So, people with dementia may begin to have trouble navigating curbs, which actually involves a number of coordinated movements, or getting in and out of cars or beds. They may just become generally clumsy. Every one, however, will eventually become less able to manipulate eating utensils and toilet paper.

■ ■ ■

These are the skills that are lost to dementia. What is much more important for us as caregivers, however, are the skills that remain.

What Isn't Lost?

Very helpful skills remain, despite dementia. You'll see this if you look for them. Recognizing and supporting the skills that remain is what makes it possible to live more comfortably with dementia and with those who are experiencing it.

The Intuitive Thought Processes

Our intuitive thought processes include some of our earliest, most primal skills as human beings. They include our ability to take in information about our surroundings using our five senses, our instantaneous and involuntary responses to those surroundings, and our ability to learn from experience. We are using intuitive thought when we have a sense about something or a feeling that we might find hard to articulate. Intuitive thought helps us see the big picture by taking in data from all our senses simultaneously, while rational thought allows us to focus on a detail. Intuitive thought causes us to startle at a loud noise, while rational thought helps us identify what the noise was. Intuitive thought is the realm of *re*action (the home of our fight-or-flight responses), while rational thought is the domain of considered action.

Functionally, our intuitive thought processes enable us to access and appreciate feelings, beauty, and sensory information. Here's what I see my clients continue to do:

Feel and interpret feelings

People with dementia know how they feel even if they can no longer name the feeling or interpret our words when we try to describe it for them. It's quite possible to feel sadness and be unable to say, "I am sad," or feel physical pain and be unable to say, "My knee hurts." It's part of being an experiential being with loss of both rational thought and language.

Recently I took a client to a medical procedure in a town several hours away. The weather was bad, long stretches of the road were under construction, the medical procedure was painful, and the clinic was crowded and noisy. My client faced one situation after another and endured a great deal of strange and unpleasant stimuli. She was exhausted and deeply confused long before we left the clinic. She turned to me and said, with tears in her eyes, "I feel like I'm floating."

I didn't say to myself, "That's the dementia talking," and ignore her statement. I knew I was with a frightened and confused woman. So, I agreed with her and expressed for her what she could not put into words—that so many confusing things had happened she couldn't possibly make sense of it, and that soon we would get into the car and head for home. That was what she needed to hear. Even if she had been unable to interpret my words, she would have been comforted by my carefully empathetic tone, facial expression, and body language.

My words validated her feelings and restored her sense of security, but she also responded to my nonverbal communication, using skills she'd learned in the cradle (not late in life). My staff and I are very careful of what we express nonverbally. Caregivers who do not realize that their charges can read how the people around them feel are unconsciously creating negative moods, exponentially increasing the emotional load on both themselves and their charges.

Enjoy beauty

When I walk into a room or garden, I can't help but feel a surge of appreciation for the symmetry of its design, textures, or colors—or be jolted by its dissymmetry. When I'm driving in town or walking in the woods, each turn exposes something new to admire. My heart leaps at first glimpse of a beautiful painting, puppy, or human face. We vary in our ability to notice and appreciate beauty, yet we can't help but have those instantaneous reactions of appreciation or antipathy when something does reach us.

I suspect that it's our rational thought processes that distract us from beauty. I've seen some of the most focused businessmen and preoccupied professors become more aware of beauty as dementia progresses. I have watched them become animated and burst into song while listening to an uplifting melody, and light up with pleasure at a YouTube video of songbirds at a snow-covered feeder.

Beauty feeds our souls, in all its forms. People with dementia respond to and benefit greatly from exposure to beauty.

Receive sensory feedback

It's our intuitive thought processes that cause us to breathe deeply when we walk outside on an early spring morning or catch the first hint of dinner cooking indoors, and the same processes that cause us to recoil from a diaper or whiff of rotting garbage. Scent is usually the first sense to be lost in dementia, followed by taste, and some people become unable to make sense of the information their optic nerves are sending to their brains. Some people lose hearing. However, the ability to receive sensory information through touch continues indefinitely.

Although people with dementia continue to receive the data their senses provide them, eventually they become unable to interpret it. One of my clients began recoiling from the passenger door when a car came up beside us in the right lane, and clinging to my arm when we walked into a noisy café. I then knew it was time for her to stay home, where we could control the amount and type of sensory stimulation she would receive.

However, for as long as the physical body is able to provide sensory data and the brain able to interpret it, caregivers can enhance their loved ones' lives with a diversity of sensory input limited only by their own imaginations.

Respond with fight or flight

When we feel threatened or at risk, we respond with fear or aggression. This part of our intuitive thought processes remains intact with dementia, too, and its effect is intensified by the lack of rational thought and memory. Frightened two-year-olds and angry teenagers are also difficult to deal with, because they also have rational thought limitations. Wise dementia caregivers go out of their way to avoid activating their charges' fight-or-flight responses.

The Experiential Self

The experiential self is an asset for someone experiencing dementia, but only if his or her caregivers recognize its existence. Our sense of what is happening now, or in the present, is everything that occurs in a span of about three seconds. That's where our companions with dementia are living.

Our experiential selves are collectors. They gather information from what surrounds us via our senses. They collect data regarding our physical environments, our companions, our own bodies. The tools they use are sight, hearing, touch, smell, and taste. How we then interpret what our experiential selves have gathered depends on our personalities, earlier life experiences, and what we believe to be true in the present.

Our interpretation of what is gathered shapes how we feel, but if we have dementia and lack memory and rational thought we will not be able to analyze and change the moods that result. People with healthy brains use recall, analysis, planning, and distraction to alter their moods; people with dementia remain trapped in their own moods and those of the people around them.

As dementia caregivers, we need to remember that when we bring negative emotions such as sorrow, concern, or frustration to our loved ones who have dementia, they absorb our moods and experience them until we introduce something more positive.

The Mindlessness Tools

Rational thought gives us the ability to focus our attention on one thing. By using prioritization, we can ignore the people talking at the next table and pay attention to what's being said at our table. We can also choose to focus our minds on the present—to feel what we're feeling, to see what's right beside us, to think about the task at hand rather than doing it while focused on something in the past or future. When we do this, we are being mindful.

Mindfulness is getting a lot of press right now, and for good reason. We miss a lot by being focused on the past or the future. However, being able to operate mind*lessly* is as beneficial for someone with dementia as being mindful is for those of us with healthy brains.

Automatic thinking scripts

When we find ourselves doing a task without thinking consciously about it, we are mindlessly using an automatic thinking script. I've made coffee so many times in my kitchen that I don't need to think about the steps while I do them. Repetition brings competency, so long as there is no alteration to the steps or the environment. Have you ever moved to a new home and caught yourself reaching for a mug in the direction it would have been in your previous home? Your mindlessness was interrupted by it not being there, but until that interruption you were using an automatic thinking script.

It is not good for those of us with healthy brains to be on autopilot, except maybe when doing mundane things like making coffee or getting dressed. But it's critically valuable to people experiencing dementia, because they cannot rely on memory to know where to look for coffee filters or socks, and they don't have rational thought to tell them that underwear goes on before pants, once memory fails.

Muscle memory

Muscle memory is how I ski moguls. My clients use muscle memory to find the bathroom in the night. I couldn't explain to you how I shift my weight, flex my muscles, or identify the fall line on a ski run because getting through a mogul field is something I do without using rational thought. My clients could never explain to you where to find the bathroom.

That's how muscle memory works. It is action specific and non-transferable. Like an automatic thinking script, the slightest change will interrupt it, which is what happens when we move people with dementia out of their homes and into care facilities. Sometimes their muscle memory leads them to a closet in the night, rather than the bathroom. When we take them away from familiarity, automatic thinking scripts, and muscle memories, they begin failing at things we thought they knew how to do. We set them adrift in an alien world.

Automatic thinking scripts and muscle memories become very valuable when someone loses memory and rational thought.

■ ■ ■

This is the pattern of abilities and disabilities I have seen my diverse dementia clientele display. When we pay attention to both the abilities and the disabilities that come with dementia, we are choosing to provide person-directed care rather than treatment.

Treatment involves identifying what's wrong and righting it. In the United States, we are very skilled at treatment. Our medical experts do an outstanding job of diagnosing symptoms, prescribing cures, and developing new treatments to deal with changing outcomes. Care is different from treatment. When we are experiencing a condition (something incurable), we must learn to live with it. We need support for both our abilities and disabilities.

Providing care means maximizing someone's quality of life through recognizing and supporting their changing abilities and disabilities. Let's now look at the best way to do that for people who have dementia.

CHAPTER 3
Designing Person-Directed Care

Once we recognize the pattern of loss and continuation that comes with dementia, we can better live with it and with the people who have it. If we understand their impairments in terms of functioning, we can choose when to do something for them and when to let them do it themselves.

Here's the pattern of what is lost and what remains with dementia:

LOST:	NOT LOST:
Rational thought	Intuitive thought
Remembering self	Experiential self
Mindfulness	Mindlessness tools

If you prefer using your rational thought processes to using your intuitive ones, you don't need to read any further in this book. Just flip back to the previous chapter and use your own analytical skills to design a care plan that takes into account the above pattern. However, if you prefer to learn by doing or are interested in how I've approached care with my clients, this chapter will summarize an approach that takes advantage of the skills I've seen my clients retain and provides support for those they are losing. The result, I've found, is that people with dementia can become happy and relaxed if they receive care that enhances their abilities. Here are the five key things we do with our clients:

Manage Mood

I manage my own mood by using memory and rational thought skills. For example, I might feel saddened when I realize I haven't heard from a friend for quite some time, but I then use memory to recall that she has just started a new job. I might use analysis to imagine the numerous new demands on her time, or cause and effect to picture her not getting home until much later each night and dozing in front of the television. I can then use analysis again to understand why I should not feel sad. Or if I have had a difficult day myself, I draw on memory and sequence to recall that I'm about to drive past Safeway on my way home and visualize the aisle where I know I will find an assortment of Ben & Jerry's ice cream. I use memory, rational thought, planning, and distraction to change my moods as I wish. If I don't choose to improve my mood right away, I still have the skills to do so later.

My clients lack those skills and are stuck with whatever feelings arise due to circumstance. Without memory, one client forgets she's just ended a phone conversation with her son who lives in a distant state and calls her every few days. She feels loss, loneliness, and abandonment standing in front of the telephone that's still warm from her touch. Another finds himself staring at the television remote, knowing that it is the key to watching the History channel and that using it was once as unconscious and easy as looking at the clock. Another sits at her kitchen table looking out of the window at her empty driveway. She is unable to recall what has happened to the blue 1972 Toyota Corolla that she remembers so vividly.

Without memory and rational thought, people who have dementia constantly experience scary and frustrating feelings they are unable to escape from. In addition, when they are with other people, they sense others' feelings and moods but are unable to deduce the reasons behind them.

Having dementia means being aware of feelings and moods without having the tools to alter them. We, as companions and caregivers, can recognize this disability and change the moods our loved ones with dementia are experiencing. If we think we are not managing their moods already, we are mistaken. When we are not actively creating positive moods for someone with dementia, we are actively allowing negative moods to develop and continue.

Remember, the good news is that because people with dementia have no tools to change their own moods, they are readily influenced by the positive moods that we bring to them.

Support Security Needs

Have you ever found yourself in a situation at work or home that gave you concern for your future security? Maybe there are more closed-door meetings going on than usual and you overheard a coworker whispering about someone being let go. Or you discovered photos on your spouse's computer quite by accident, photos that force you to question his or her commitment to your marriage. Once doubt creeps in, a sense of security is very difficult to recapture. You can still be happy from time to time, but any lasting sense of happiness or well-being has been extinguished along with trust.

When people begin to experience dementia—as memory falters and fails, and rational thought processes become intermittent and then elusive—any sense of security evaporates. There is nothing scarier than realizing that you can no longer trust your brain to correctly interpret the world around you or supply you with accurate information. Even when people are unaware of how impaired they are, they seem to know their futures are at risk. Living with worsening forgetfulness and confusion and knowing that you will become completely unable to care for yourself is rightfully terrifying.

People experiencing dementia need help in recovering a sense of security before they can recapture any lasting sense of well-being. Unless their caregivers and loved ones show them that they can still be safe despite dementia, that ever-so-necessary sense of comfort in the day-to-day routines of life will be fleeting.

We help our clients begin to feel secure even though they are confused, because we use our own rational thought skills when analysis is necessary, and we use our own memories to supply the gaps in theirs. When they ask questions, we remind ourselves that although they have lost the ability to retain information, they still need to know what's going on as much as we do. We never jog their memories, knowing that testing memory only serves to prove and prove again that they've lost the ability to remember, not just the memories themselves.

We also help them find what they've misplaced or complete a task without ever saying, "I've already told you" or "I can't believe you don't remember that." When we offer help as an equal and teammate, rather than a superior or instructor, our clients' dignity and sense of autonomy remain intact. There is no loss of control or hurt feelings. With our own rational thought skills, we foresee the next step in a task and work with them rather than direct them.

Further, as their sense of reality becomes increasingly divergent from ours, we accept it as the inevitable result of progressive cognitive impairment and accommodate it, rather than demand that they use skills that no longer exist. While we are doing this, our clients begin to relax and feel secure in the knowledge (through experiential learning while with us) that we will take care of them despite their growing needs and escalating confusion.

Enhance Well-Being

Someone who does not have a sense that life is good and all is well is at least uncomfortable and more probably distressed. Being distressed affects how we interpret what's going on around us and how we respond. It heightens the fight-or-flight response.

My clients seem to experience distress in four key areas as they progress through dementia: social interactions, autonomy, sense of worth, and view of the future. When their caregivers and companions help them in these four areas, they recover the sense of well-being that is so elusive with dementia. Recovering well-being means regaining peace of mind, which leads to more comfort and companionship. Here are the principal well-being needs that my clients exhibit:

Social success

When someone is experiencing dementia, social success is as simple as being able to interact with others without embarrassment or conflict. Memory loss affects every interaction, no matter how casual. When we converse, whether with people we know, with strangers, or while conducting business, we assume an array of known facts. When I chatted with my mother the other night on the phone, one part of our conversation went like this:

"So, have you heard anything?"

"Nope, nothing this week. Have you? Carolyn said she got an e-mail."

"I wonder if he met up with Mandy."

"She didn't say. Are you sending his present the same way as last year?"

"Probably, unless I hear otherwise. But what'd he say about work?"

"Not much. I don't think it's a problem, though. Internet cafés are everywhere."

"Well, that's good. At least he's safer there than he was during the coup."

Although you can't assume much more than that we're talking about a family member, my mother and I both knew exactly who and what we were talking about, because we both have memory at our disposal. We knew we were talking about my son who works via the Internet, was living in Turkey last summer, and is spending the winter traveling in Asia. None of those facts were stated. If my mother develops dementia, however, our conversations will be very different. I will have to restate all the supporting facts as we converse so that she can follow along without recall.

Likewise, when someone stands at a grocery-store checkout or teller's window, the conversation is based on a broad array of assumptions—from the meaning of "cash or credit" to the ability to deduce whether a piece of paper represents a request for payment or a statement of assets. Someone experiencing dementia will need a companion who restates what the rest of us would consider obvious. Without that kind of support, confusion and embarrassment are inevitable.

It is memory that would inform the husband in the first chapter that when his wife says, "We need to go to Safeway," she wants to buy groceries. Without memory, his first question upon hearing that statement is likely to be, "Why?" He would be asking, "Why is Safeway a place we need to go?" It's a valid question for someone without memory.

If she has typically responded to such questions in the past, however, with exasperation or affront (because she assumes he's being difficult, not lacking in memory), he's not likely to ask. He is more likely to simply say no, meaning, "I don't know what you're talking about, so I prefer to avoid further embarrassment by refusing." Without rational thought skills, such as cause and effect, he also won't know that buying groceries would replenish their supply of Oreos and his breakfast cereal, or enable her to make his favorite meatloaf for dinner that night.

Without the information that memory and recall provide, we are easily embarrassed and fail in our human relationships. The caregiver who assumes memory and rational thought loss will enhance social success rather than destroy it.

Sense of control

Choice is addictive. Children start out with little of it, but with each bit obtained strive to acquire more of it from their parents, some sooner and more strenuously than others. By the time we reach adulthood, we are accustomed to being able to make numerous choices daily, from what shirt to wear, to how to get downtown, to whether to purchase a Ford or Prius. When rational thought fails, however, we begin making poorer choices. Keep in mind, though, that the failure of rational thought and good decision making does not negate the desire to exercise autonomy. People with dementia still need to feel in control of themselves and their lives.

Wise caregivers recognize this as an opportunity to develop and maintain well-being and companionship. Recalling that her husband prefers Oreos over oatmeal-raisin cookies and coffee over tea—knowing that he is losing vocabulary, the ability to track time, and maybe also the ability to recognize hunger—the wife above could ask, "Would you like a cup of coffee and an Oreo?" rather than, "Do you feel like having a snack?" She would be using her own memory and rational thought on his behalf, while offering him choices.

Framing choices as either/or questions or single-option questions extends autonomy, as does making something visible. The family of one of our clients reported that he often refused to use the bathroom. Rather than assume that he was being difficult or belligerent, we assumed that he had a problem with memory and rational thought. My caregiver simply asked him if he'd like to come down the hall with her to look in the mirror. He was happy to do that; it sounded interesting. Once he looked into the bathroom, he saw the toilet, which stimulated the sensation of needing to use it. He wasn't exercising autonomy in choosing to not use the bathroom when asked. He was exercising his lack of vocabulary, failing ability to interpret sensations, and nonexistent understanding of cause and effect.

My caregivers and I see the drawback in our clients' loss of rational thought, but we also see the advantage it gives us in preserving them from their own flawed judgment. This touches on the much larger topic of the difference between motivating people and manipulating them. Rest assured that if your intentions are for the good of the other person, not yourself, you are being motivational, not manipulative.

When our clients are acting against their own interests or needs, we present the activity to them as if it were their own idea, or we draw their focus to individual steps rather than the end goal. So, rather than tell my client, "You need to go to the doctor to have that toe looked at," I might say, "You asked me if I'd go with you to your doctor today—I'd be glad to." And if she still adamantly refuses, I can invite her out for coffee and a drive. Once she's in the car, she's likely to be willing to accompany me on an errand (which happens to be visiting her doctor's office) and will probably choose to come in with me rather than wait in the car. As long as I don't say, "You must come with me to this doctor's appointment," we have a good chance of ending up in an exam room where a friendly nurse can examine the infected toe.

We, as caregivers, can use our own memory and rational thought to enhance our loved ones' autonomy and safety, despite their cognitive losses.

Sense of value

We all need to be needed, to have something to contribute, and to have relationships in which we play an active role. One of the most debilitating aspects of life in a traditional American care facility is that residents have no chores, no purpose, no connection with the outside community—no means of doing anything of value for someone else. They are constantly the recipients of assistance, not givers of anything. The overly efficient caregiver spouse or child causes the same disempowerment. Yet people need to be able to contribute and to give, whether dementia is in the picture or not. Care facility residents thrive and their disabilities diminish when they have pets to care for, or even just a potted plant to water.

When I allow my client to make choices and take part in the tasks of daily life, I am being respectful and giving him or her the ability to play a role. When I listen for the message hidden behind fading language skills, I am enabling equality. I can use my own memory and rational thought to make it possible for both of us to contribute to our common needs and goals. My client can then retain a sense of self-worth.

Hopefully, I can offer my clients admiration and love, not just respect. Although we cannot always offer all three, at the very least we can offer respect for their personhood by recognizing their abilities as well as their disabilities.

Ram Dass said, "We're all just walking each other home." To me, that expresses the relationship between a dementia caregiver and care receiver perfectly. The two are equals. Both have strengths, just different ones. Both need help, in dissimilar ways. Working together, they each experience more quality of life.

Secure future

I look around at my family, friends, and colleagues and see security symbols everywhere. One grew up poor and decided that the secret to a good life lay in becoming a doctor or attorney. Now close to retiring from a career as a law professor, he gets great satisfaction from the size of his retirement accounts. Another finds future security in church attendance and her faith; another feels security in becoming a member of a prestigious club and forming friendships there. My own sense of security comes from owning a home.

My clients are no different, except that their personal security symbols seem to become truncated and simplified as their dementia proceeds. One woman who found security in having large account balances became fixated on daily visits to the bank to have a teller verify that her savings were still intact. That was a logical and predictable behavior for someone who lacked memory and found security in her bank accounts.

We began congratulating her on how smart she and her husband had been to save so much money, on their wisdom in choosing such a secure bank, on how lucky she was to have such a business-wise son to help her preserve her assets. After a few weeks of reminders that her future security was ensured in the manner that mattered to her, she lost the need for those daily bank visits. We had helped her regain the sense that her future was safe.

Our security symbols are real—they enable us to look forward without trepidation. When dementia begins affecting memory and rational thought, our symbols might become skewed or nonsensical, but the need to know that we are equipped to meet the future remains. The caregiver who validates a loved one's security symbol enables well-being.

Look for Beauty

Beauty is food for the soul. It feeds and supports our humanity. I don't think I ever saw one of my horses look out a stall door to admire a sunset or my dog pause to savor the fragrance of a violet. But something within us as humans responds to beauty in all its forms.

We have five ways to enjoy beauty. We can see, hear, touch, smell, or taste it. Our need to encounter beauty in as many forms as possible, and our response to it, does not disappear when dementia arrives. In my clients, it seems to intensify.

As caregivers of people experiencing dementia, if we are not actively looking for beauty to bring into our loved ones' awareness, we are actively denying them of it. They are becoming ever less able to seek it out for themselves. Music is a way to enjoy beauty that is particularly effective with people who have dementia, for a number of reasons. I have a friend who loves jazz. Now that she has dementia, she cannot go the stereo and put on her Dave Brubeck CD and listen to him play "Take Five." Without her friends' help, she would never again hear Miles Davis, Ella Fitzgerald, or John Coltrane. We must actively bring her beauty in the forms that speak to her.

Beauty is everywhere—in sounds, flavors, colors, textures, and scents. The smallest dose can soothe, satisfy, even revitalize. As caregivers, it's our duty to identify and bring what works to the people we work with.

Manage Stimulation

Our need for stimulation—both sensory and social—does not end when dementia appears. I shudder when I walk through a care facility and see people slumped in wheelchairs in hallways, alone in rooms with nothing but a bed and television, or at the table being fed overcooked and lukewarm meals. If my family were to check me into a care facility, I would be exhibiting negative behaviors within twenty-four hours, due to lack of stimulation.

Just as surely as our stomachs need food, our brains need the stimulation provided by new sensory data, but more continuously. When either organ doesn't get what it needs, discomfort results. If your loved one with dementia isn't sleeping at night or is restless by late afternoon, evaluate how much stimulation he or she is getting during the day. An unstimulated brain is a restless brain and a demanding one.

We try to get our clients outside. Fresh air does wonders for children, adults, and elders. If the weather won't let us stay outside long, we head for the mall. We savor lattes or protein smoothies and do some people watching. We wander the teen boutiques and feel the texture of the T-shirts decorated with sequins and fringes. We marvel at the color of shoes or the height of their heels; we admire racks of buttons and bolts of calico in the fabric store. Or we drive to the hardware store, where there are bins of nails, aisles of bedding plants, walls of paint chips—countless opportunities to stimulate our clients' senses.

Find errands to run together. Even the grocery store is stocked with beauty and sensory stimulation; if you look for it, you will see it. Point it out and stop to savor it. Have you ever noticed how pretty a pineapple is? It's also heavy, and both smooth and rough. It's sticky and prickly, and it smells good. Take advantage of sensory stimulation where you can find it.

Social stimulation is just as important, but in varying ways. We consider how introverted or extroverted our clients were earlier in life, although that sometimes changes as dementia progresses. For those who are extroverts and thrive in groups and meetings, a quiet afternoon at home can be distressing. For an introvert, it's likely to be restorative. We take our cues from our clients as to what forms of social stimulation to offer.

People who have dementia need stimulation, both sensory and social. They can't pursue it themselves, but we can actively bring it to them.

■ ■ ■

This is a brief description of how my caregivers and I provide care that maximizes our clients' quality of life, despite dementia, by supporting their changing abilities and disabilities. My second book, *Dementia with Dignity*, details the tools and techniques my caregivers and I use. This approach, which I developed with our clients at the Dementia & Alzheimer's Wellbeing Network® (DAWN), has come to be known as the DAWN Method. It's habilitative in philosophy and person-directed in approach.

CHAPTER 4

Person-Directed Care in Action

The previous chapter described the five essential needs that my caregivers and I have found must be addressed for our clients to understand that they are safe and to develop a sense that all is well from one day to the next, even though they are experiencing the continued decline in abilities caused by dementia. Now, let's look at putting the techniques and tools of the DAWN Method to use in specific situations.

Keep in mind that while dementia eventually leads to complete loss of rational thought and memory, these losses occur over time. Your loved one is on a continuum of decline, experiencing a gradual and sometimes quite sudden loss of abilities. We need to tailor our assistance to match our loved ones' current mix of ability and disability. Too much care too soon will be perceived as offensive and demeaning. Remember that our goal in all interactions with people who have dementia is to preserve their dignity and autonomy to the greatest extent possible and for as long as possible.

These situational excerpts are drawn from the Caregiver Tips that I write for the DAWN Method website.

■ ■ ■

Dementia and the Calendar

How to Help Your Loved One Feel on Top of Things

When dementia strikes, one of the most disconcerting losses is becoming unable to track time, understand the calendar, or keep appointments.

Can you remember an occasion when you struggled to understand a concept, and then suddenly, comprehension dawned? As we progressed through childhood, we daily enjoyed that welcome rush of understanding—of mastery of an idea or the way to do something. As adults, however, we are so accustomed to understanding what we see, read, and hear that we forget how frustrating and scary it is not to be able to do so. If you have traveled in a country where you did not speak the language, you have had a reminder of how it feels to be unable to make sense of what you see or hear.

When people are experiencing dementia, they are traveling in a land that is becoming increasingly foreign to them. Hard as it is to be unable to interpret information, they are also becoming unable to imagine how quickly the clock hand moves from 12:00 to 12:05 or how much longer it will take to move from 12:05 to 3:00. Further, they are becoming unable to hold two facts in their minds at once, unable to see cause and effect, unable to make plans, and unable to initiate activities for themselves.

With these skills fading or gone, how can we expect them to calmly accept an assertion that it is time to go to an appointment or that we can go out for breakfast and be back to meet a friend by noon?

The inability to perceive the passage of time or read clocks or calendars becomes a constant cause of stress for caregivers. How can we enhance our loved ones' ability to track time and feel more comfortable with deadlines? Here are a few tips based on what we do with our clients at DAWN.

Accept 'possible' and give up 'probable'

Experiencing dementia means losing rational thought processes but keeping the intuitive ones, so people become unable to learn through memorizing or reasoning but continue to learn from experience. If we were to let keeping appointments become a source of conflict, we would begin to see difficult behaviors escalating around time issues. Instead, we keep in mind that when someone has dementia, it is always *possible* that we will make it to an appointment on time, but never *probable*.

In addition, we focus our attention on our clients, not on the deadline, and on no more than one preparatory task at a time. When we do this, the probability of being able to make the deadline or keep the appointment increases. More importantly, however, our clients learn that it is fun to do things with us rather than learning that we become agitated when a deadline is looming.

Keep it simple

We use large calendars that show no more than one month when laid open on the counter. Each morning, we cross out the day before so that the first square not crossed out is always today. We watch to see whether our clients are better at interpreting times as 3 *p.m.*, *3:00*, or 3 *o'clock* and use that format only. We always note activities with the time first and follow the time with a succinct description of the event. We use white out rather than crossing out changes or mistakes. In addition, we place notepaper and a pen nearby so they can write their own notes, because writing something out gives a feeling of mastery and security.

Schedule one activity per day

When our clients are in the early stages of dementia, they are able to manage more than one activity in a day without becoming stressed. As their dementia progresses, we cut their activities back to one each morning and afternoon and then to one per day. Eventually, we focus on providing appropriate sensory and social stimulation in brief interactions rather than lengthier activities.

Helping clients to feel safe even though they cannot read the clock or make sense of the passage of time is an important way to provide support as dementia caregivers.

■ ■ ■

Dementia and the Conversation

How do we help people with dementia take part in conversations successfully? We use several simple techniques to help our clients avoid embarrassment, join in conversations, and contribute successfully when they are in a group.

Be the supplier of fact

We start by cheerfully stating the obvious. Have you ever thought about how much information we assume our listeners already know when we converse? If I were to bump into a friend in the grocery store, she might ask me, "How'd that go last Friday?" or "When does Jean get home?" If I go into the bank with a question about an account, the teller might say, "Yes, that information will be on your statement." A lot of known information is assumed in these interactions.

People with dementia are becoming ever less able to recall facts or events and may have forgotten the meaning of words such as *account.* Statements like the ones above leave them bewildered and unable to continue without asking questions about things that seem obvious to those of us with healthy brains. When we are with our clients, we are careful to state and restate any necessary background facts—cheerfully.

Focus on the present

When we are alone with our clients, we want them to enjoy companionable conversation with us. We start by choosing topics from what is there in our presence. We avoid bringing up events from the near past and future, which would require memory and rational thought to discuss. Instead, we look around; anything we can see, hear, taste, smell, or touch is good subject matter. People with dementia are able to enjoy sensory information through their intuitive thought processes, so we turn to what is nearby for the subject matter of our conversations.

Become a spectator

Sitting in a coffee shop, restaurant, park, or shopping mall provides a constantly changing array of people to watch. People—especially children—and pets provide valuable entertainment. Several years ago, I had a client who could not get over the price of clothing, especially what was being charged for jeans with holes in them. It delighted her to sit at the Starbucks in the mall and watch the students wander by in their trendy ragged jeans and then join me in exclaiming over price tags in clothing shops on our way out.

Encourage favorite anecdotes

We all have favorite stories or jokes we love to tell. For some reason, certain anecdotes just make us feel good. Why is it embarrassing when we catch ourselves repeating one and irritating when someone else does it? We need to remember that people experiencing dementia cannot help repeating themselves.

With our clients, we accept repetition as a condition of dementia and, instead of feeling frustrated or bored when our clients launch into the same tale yet again, we prompt them to retell it at least once every time we are with them. When they tell it, we listen attentively and respond as if we have never heard it before. We know that expressing our enjoyment at their story or joke is a gift that we can give them.

Introduce forgotten memories

When people have dementia, it is unkind to put them on the spot and expect them to use memory skills they are losing or have already lost. It is a great kindness, however, to recount for them the memories we know they once loved and drew great enjoyment from recalling. We are our clients' storytellers. We tell them their memories as if we are narrating much-loved bedtime stories.

The best part about spending time with someone who has dementia and using the techniques I describe above is that it is refreshing. It requires us to use our own intuitive thought processes, which is a release from the constant demands on rational thought required by navigating daily life in a technological world. So, enjoy yourself. Look for beauty and stimulation. It will enhance your own sense of well-being as well as your companion's.

■ ■ ■

Dementia and the Dinner Table

Does your loved one have issues with food, eating, or mealtime? We do a number of things at DAWN to make mealtimes easier.

Our first step is always to look for an underlying emotional need. Any behavioral problem is likely to be the result of feelings of disempowerment, embarrassment, confusion, or risk. If we can identify an emotional problem, we meet that need first. Once we have ruled out or taken care of emotional needs, we watch for a few additional things.

Failure to recognize hunger

People experiencing dementia may lose the ability to feel hunger or to interpret and understand what to do about that feeling. However, rather than telling our clients that they need to eat or should eat, we invite them to eat with us, saying that we feel hungry or we prefer to eat with them. We do not want them to feel awkward eating alone while we stand by.

In addition, while we are preparing the meal, we ask them to sample tidbits and help us decide how much salt is needed or whether something is hot enough—anything we can think of to involve them in preparation and sneak in a little extra nutrition. These approaches enhance companionship and allow our clients to help us—a welcome change from always being the person in need.

Too much on the plate

When someone routinely refuses to eat, we switch to a brightly colored plate and are careful not to overload it. We place small servings of each item on the plate, separating them so that the plate is visible between them. I have often had clients refuse to eat from a heaped plate, saying they couldn't possibly eat that much. Scarcity seems to enhance appeal.

Vision problems

Be sure to have your loved one's eyes checked for issues such as cataracts or macular degeneration. However, sometimes even though a person's vision is not impaired, his or her brain fails to interpret the information being sent by the optic nerve. We find that when people seem unresponsive to food that is in front of them, pointing to the item or moving the item will sometimes make it seeable and prompt them to eat it.

Utensil problems

We should expect our loved ones and clients eventually to forget what eating utensils are and how to use them. When this happens, we model use of the fork, spoon, or knife. When modeling stops being helpful, we begin presenting foods in mouthful-sized pieces that can be eaten with the fingers. While we are eating together with our clients, we talk about what we are eating and how good it tastes.

Too much commotion

As people progress deeper into dementia, it becomes more difficult for them to interpret sensory stimulation. This means that when there is background music or television, several people talking at once, or lots of coming and going from the table, people with dementia are less able to focus on eating. We gauge our clients' ability to handle stimuli and modify the environment to meet their current levels of functioning.

Hydrate!

The symptoms of dehydration can mimic dementia. We are always looking for ways to get more fluids into our clients' routines. We find a beverage they like to drink and offer it often. Poor nutrition, low blood sugar, and dehydration all make people physically uncomfortable, and physical discomfort is expressed in behaviors.

■ ■ ■

Dementia and Finding Those Missing Keys

People who have dementia lose things constantly. It is a tremendous source of stress for them as well as for their caregivers, housekeepers, friends, and family members. When a person can't recall what happened a few minutes ago, let alone this morning, it can seem likely to her that someone took her wallet or hairbrush. And, with dementia in the picture, more often than not, the missing item will eventually be found someplace very odd.

How do we help someone who is distressed about losing something? We face this issue almost daily. Our response is to take our client's focus off the problem—the *absence* of the item—and help him or her focus on the process of finding it.

We never get upset. Losing things is an unavoidable part of dementia. There are two primary benefits of focusing on the search rather than reacting with frustration and joining in our clients' panic over the loss.

Building teamwork and de-emphasizing mastery

People experiencing dementia are becoming ever less able to accomplish tasks or solve problems on their own. Losing competency is very distressing. We spend our entire lives becoming masters at tasks, activities, and problem solving. Children gradually acquire the skills needed to perform their own personal hygiene tasks, feed themselves, and follow directions. They grow older and drive cars, navigate the education system, and become more tech-savvy than their parents are. They learn to cook, mow the lawn, find a good mechanic, and order takeout. The list of daily tasks that we master as residents of a technological world is endless.

Dementia takes away these abilities one by one. When we repeatedly fail, we eventually give up and retreat into passivity. So, dementia requires a teammate—someone who will help you learn to give up being a master and accept needing a partner to accomplish tasks. Searching for something together is an excellent way to collaborate in solving a problem, so long as the caregiver keeps the focus on the *process* of finding the item.

Relief in following a process

If I am missing my purse or hearing aid or glasses, I have a big problem. Something essential or valuable is beyond my reach, so I am distressed. However, if I have dementia as well, I have an even bigger problem. I am missing the two tools I most need to solve my first problem: memory and the rational thought skills that would help me to form a plan or follow a series of steps. I will be unable to arrive at a place where I can say to myself, "Well, I've done everything I can do to find it. It will eventually turn up. I can turn my attention to something else now."

If I am with someone who will collaborate with me and lead me through the process of searching, my first problem will likely be solved. A systematic search usually turns up missing items. More importantly, having someone partner with me will keep me from repeatedly internalizing the feeling of being out of control and at risk. There is a degree of success and control in being able to take steps and follow a process.

We, as caregivers, need to give our loved ones and clients the sense of success that comes from following processes. When we lead them—without getting angry or worried—through a systematic search for whatever is missing, we turn an episode of panic into an opportunity to learn that there is safety and empowerment in partnership.

At DAWN, when something goes missing, we welcome the chance to be teammates with our clients and help them avoid the passivity that results from experiencing constant failure.

■ ■ ■

Dementia and the Grocery Store

Running errands with someone who has dementia can be very trying. We can do two things to make it easier. It really does not matter where we need to take our clients—the grocery store, bank, hardware store, or a utility company—we avoid behaviors and have a companionable time by looking at errands as an opportunity to find sensory and social stimulation.

Search Out the Beautiful

It's here. It's there. It's everywhere. If you are looking, there is beauty at every turn. The florist department may seem like the only place in a grocery store to find something pretty, but if you are in the produce department, pick up any piece of fruit and look. It is colorful, intricate, and, if not beautiful, at least interesting. Are you searching for a particular variety of soup? Look closely at the labels; the photos on cans and boxes are often pleasing to the eye. Are you shopping for cheese? The shiny red packaging of a Gouda or bright orange of cheddar is very appealing.

Look for colors and patterns, good smells and textures. In a hardware store, there is a myriad of sights and smells—displays of paint chips and bins of drawer pulls. In offices, there are calendars, plants on people's desks, interesting gadgets. We are always on the lookout for something that will provide our clients with new sensory stimulation.

We treat every errand as a treasure hunt—a search for something new or pleasing. People with dementia retain the ability to recognize beauty. We can enjoy it with them. When we do, errands become opportunities for companionship.

In addition to using errands as an opportunity to get much-needed stimulation, we again use the technique of focusing on the person rather than on the task.

Focus on the Person and Not on the Task

As people progress deeper into dementia, the ability to track the passage of time fades. People experiencing dementia become increasingly limited to what is known as the psychological present, which lasts about three seconds. Without the ability to use rational thought functions, such as planning or foresight, or the ability to grasp cause and effect, people with dementia are living in a moment that can feel as if it lasts an eternity.

What this means for us, as caregivers, is that it becomes essential that our loved ones and clients perceive us to be focused on them and not on a task or deadline. If our goal is to have a good time with them, their experience will be that of doing something enjoyable with a person who appreciates them. If our goal is to run an errand or meet a deadline, their experience will be abandonment and disempowerment. When the latter occurs, behaviors result.

Here at DAWN, we have found that if we are communicating to our clients that we enjoy being with them, we can accomplish any task more easily. It may sound counterintuitive, but focusing on your loved one is your best chance to succeed at running an errand, making a deadline, or accomplishing a task.

. . .

Dementia and Masking

How to Avoid Being Kept in the Dark

Most parents are hesitant about letting their children know that they lost the car at the grocery store yesterday or burned a pot on the stove the day before, whether cognitive issues have been diagnosed or not. How do we keep communications open and honest with a loved one who may be experiencing the onset of dementia?

Typically, when people are experiencing memory and rational thought losses, they go to great lengths to hide their cognitive decline. It is embarrassing to forget names or get details wrong in conversation, so they try to be vague. Too many failures at self-care or instances of confusion bring concern and interference from family and friends, so they begin to isolate themselves. Masking failures gives someone with dementia a false sense of security from change, so most go to great lengths to hide problems. Yet masking prevents caregivers from preserving safety and providing targeted assistance.

When we know which tasks and areas our loved ones need help with, we can better protect their dignity and autonomy. So, how can we help someone experiencing dementia be more open about his or her increasing needs?

Here are a few strategies we use with our clients that encourage them not to hide their growing limitations from us.

Don't react emotionally when you discover something of concern

When we react with concern, fear, or anger, the message we deliver is adversarial rather than supportive. It communicates the threat of change, and no one welcomes being pressured or forced to make changes. We all treasure our autonomy, whether we have dementia or not.

Instead, you might say, "Mom, that's worrisome. I'll bet that scared you. Let's think about a way to fix things so that doesn't happen again. I know you really want to stay home." Joining with a loved one in problem solving will lower the likelihood that she will mask confusion and memory loss. It will also build trust in you as a care partner—someone who will be a teammate in preserving her independence and autonomy in safe ways.

Be empathetic

It is far too easy to be critical when a loved one loses the keys or cannot remember where to find the coffee filters, but empathetic responses to forgetfulness and confusion are essential if we want the person experiencing dementia to trust us with proof of failing abilities. Becoming more forgetful is also a part of natural aging, so we should be able to respond with patience and understanding.

Destigmatize forgetfulness

It is no fun always being the person who cannot keep up in conversation, who forgets things and loses track of time, who can never figure out what is going on. So, be open about your own instances of forgetfulness or clumsiness. Lose your keys on the table in front of him so he can find them for you. Claim fault for forgetting that medical appointment instead of pointing out that she said she would write it down. Destigmatizing forgetfulness and confusion is another way we can be partners rather than superiors in the care relationship.

As caregivers, our job is to find the balance between our charges' safety and their selfhood. We provide targeted care to preserve safety, while looking for every possible way to support personal preferences and autonomy.

■ ■ ■

Dementia and Mistaken Identities

Help! Dad Thinks I'm Mom!

When a loved one with dementia stops recognizing us, or responds to us as if we are someone else, it can be both disconcerting and hurtful. However, it is important that we understand what may have caused our loved one to believe we are someone else. When we understand the changes in cognition and perception of reality that occur with dementia, it is less painful to deal with mistaken identities.

He's living in the past

We know that dementia takes away memory, but do we understand that losing short-term memory can move a person's psychological present ever deeper into the past? With the dementia that results from Alzheimer's disease in particular, people lose all of their most recent memories first, so that although they cannot recall the near past, they do recall the distant past. This means that they also lose knowledge of the appearance of their loved ones, as it has changed over the years. When knowledge of the past is being wiped out starting with today, then yesterday, then all of last week, last month, and last year, it causes the person's belief of where he is in life to recede ever deeper into the past.

If your father's perception of the present is now twenty or thirty years in the past, he may see in your face the woman who was his wife and your mother in her earlier years. He also expects you to be the little girl he remembers from that time.

He's forgotten what you look like

We know that people experiencing dementia stop recognizing their friends and loved ones as they progressively lose the ability to recall facts and the rational thought process of forming associations. But it may also happen because dementia is affecting the area of the brain that enables us to recognize features and familiarity in human faces.

All of us have varying degrees of expertise in facial recognition. In Britain, Scotland Yard employs a special unit of *superrecognizers* who can recognize criminals or terrorists in grainy video footage even though they may be wearing ski masks. Most of us do not have that level of facial-recognition skill, but dementia can affect that area of our brains and take away whatever skills we once had.

You sound like your mom

Although people experiencing dementia lose the ability to make associations and recall faces, the ability to recognize voices seems to last longer. We often find that our clients will not immediately recognize family members when they walk in the door even though they know them when talking to them on the telephone. After a minute or two, we will see our clients warm up, perhaps because they recognize voices by using the same skills used to recognize and recall music.

In any case, when you greet your father or telephone him, he may hear your mother's tone and intonation in your voice and so mistake you for her even though you do not look familiar to him.

How should we respond?

The most important thing is to avoid reacting with concern or hurt. Becoming unable to recognize our loved ones is part of experiencing dementia. We should grieve in private and respond to our loved ones with calm acceptance or redirection. You might be able to say, "Oh, Mom's not here yet, but she's coming later." However, if redirection does not work, it is usually best simply to accept the mistaken identity.

One of our clients came home from a family event convinced that his son was in fact his brother. It did not matter that the two men had lived their lives at the opposite ends of the country, were very different in personality and age, or even that the brother had died. Our client's belief that his son was his brother never changed. We all simply accepted this new identity designation and encouraged his love and admiration for both men.

■ ■ ■

Dementia and the Telephone

How do I talk on the phone with Mom now that she has dementia? We baby boomers are a very mobile generation. Not many of us live in the same city or town we grew up in, which means that most of us are trying to stay in touch with aging parents who live far enough away that we cannot simply drop by to see how they are.

For many families, the primary means of contact is still the telephone, because using Skype and Facetime are newer skills. When a parent is experiencing dementia or even mild cognitive impairment, having a good phone conversation becomes difficult. How can we have positive phone experiences with someone who has dementia?

Of course, we expect that due to memory loss, people with dementia will have trouble bringing to mind what they did earlier that day, let alone what has happened during the past week. And we know that how much they can remember will diminish as time goes on. At first, you may find that you can ask leading questions by including a fact or two. ("Dad, did you have coffee with your friend George this morning?") During the earlier stages, memories might become available through prompting.

We need to keep in mind, however, that recalling events eventually will become impossible. We also need to remember that people with dementia often become unable to distinguish between dreamed events and real events. A parent may tell us that something happened when it was actually part of a dream. We need to be careful not to react as if he is purposefully trying to mislead us.

Avoid fact-finding

When on the phone, our purpose should be to communicate our desire to spend time with him—to express love and caring rather than to gather information. We should not expect factual information from someone who is losing memory and rational thought. What someone with dementia says has happened is possibly true but not necessarily true. So, do not correct him or question the validity of what he says. Focus on what matters: communicating that you enjoy talking with him.

Brighten her day

Treat a phone call as your chance to brighten your parent's day. When she becomes unable to recall her own experiences, use your calls as a chance to tell her what you have been doing during the past week. Recall and retell a favorite memory from your childhood or a time spent together that you know was a happy time for her, too. Use your phone call to sing songs with your mom or tell her stories of things she did that enriched your life. Your goal should be to give your loved one the experience of having your full attention and love by recalling happy times that he or she cannot recall independently.

Prepare before dialing

Before you call, write down several incidents from your own week that you know your parent will enjoy hearing about. You will be able to stay on the phone longer, avoid awkward pauses, and truly communicate that you want to spend time with him or her. Every time he or she returns to asking about the weather or how you are, take that as a cue to share another anecdote. When someone with dementia does this, she is trying to keep the conversation going; she is *not* communicating a lack of interest. It is not an indication that she was not listening but rather that she has lost memory skills.

Most importantly, remember that moods last longer for people who have dementia than for those of us with healthy brains. If you take care of providing the stories and anecdotes for your conversation, your loved one will experience companionship and love and not feel that he has failed at a conversation. He will retain the sense of being loved long after you hang up.

■ ■ ■

How to Enable Choice, Not Restrict It

People experiencing dementia are losing the ability to use recall, which, when combined with rational thought loss, makes decision making increasingly difficult. To make a choice, we must first bring to mind the available options. Next, we grade the options for such things as preference, availability, and maybe easiness or cost—all while retaining each possibility in our minds. All of this happens in a second or two, but going through the process is necessary every time we want to exercise choice.

Think, for instance, of what you might do when lunchtime draws near and you begin to feel hungry. Assuming that you recognized hunger (a skill often lost in dementia) and then decided to eat lunch and headed for the kitchen, you need to know where to find the options. We see our clients gradually lose the knowledge that cupboards open or that they contain food. They eventually stop recognizing refrigerators or, when they look inside, they see cartons and containers but fail to understand that those are sources of food.

Memory and rational thought losses have a tremendous impact on one's ability to make decisions. How can we help our loved ones retain autonomy for as long as possible?

Make options visible

Putting clothing or food out where your loved one will see it is a great way to help him or her exercise choice. We lay out items of clothing on the bed in the order they should be put on and then offer help only if necessary. When clients start losing understanding of packaging and cupboards, we set out fruit and snacks on the counter. We put a plate of food on the table with a glass of water so that when a client walks by, food and drink are visible, and he or she can choose whether to partake. Eventually, more help will be needed, but making objects or options visible is an effective means of prolonging autonomy.

Use either/or questions

Avoid using open-ended questions. When you ask people with dementia, "What would you like to do?" you are asking them to use rational thought and memory. They must bring to mind options and evaluate them. The kinder approach is to present the options in either/or style. "Would you like to eat here or go out?" That question could be followed by, "Okay, out sounds good to me, too. Which sounds better—sushi or a hamburger?" Then, once you are in the car, offer another option. "We could get hamburgers at Wendy's or Zip's. Your choice."

Eventually, selecting from two options will become too much. At that point, put the choice you think your loved one would most enjoy at the end of the sentence. So, if you know she prefers sushi, ask whether she would like to go out for "hamburgers or sushi." The last word heard will be most likely to elicit a response. A time also will come when it is best to offer only one choice: "Would you like to go out for sushi?"

Keep in mind that although the memory and rational thought losses of dementia take away a person's ability to consider options and exercise choice, the desire and need for control over one's life and body remain intact. As caregivers, we should actively look for ways to preserve and enhance our loved one's sense of autonomy. After all, when someone feels powerless, the quickest way to regain a sense of control is to refuse to cooperate and, without rational thought, refusals often put safety at risk.

Enhancing our clients and loved ones' ability to exercise choice and feel autonomous is another way we can show them love and respect.

■ ■ ■

How to Give the Gift of Giving

The DAWN Method is an approach that teaches caregivers to look for the emotional needs that lead to behaviors for people who have dementia. We teach caregivers to recognize and meet their loved ones' security needs first, so they can feel safe even though they are confused, need others to care for them, and cannot manage their own moods. We also teach caregivers to enhance their charges' sense of well-being. One of the essential components of well-being is to feel valued—to have a role and be needed and appreciated in relationships. When dementia strikes, keeping this intact takes conscious effort on the caregiver's part.

Being able to give gifts can be an important aspect of feeling a sense of value. Eventually, as dementia progresses, the awareness of gift giving will diminish, but until it does, we need to help our loved ones feel successful in expressing love and generosity.

Make choosing gifts easier

When someone is losing memory and rational thought, keeping track of dates, names, and facts becomes increasingly difficult. As caregivers, we should take care of these functions. You might begin by sitting down together and compiling a list of the people your loved one would like to give something to, then identifying what that would be for each person.

Reserve the actual purchasing for another day. Go shopping together, list in hand, and address one person at a time, checking off each name as you go. Treat finding each gift as a separate task that can be successfully completed. It will probably be best to tackle the list on more than one day.

We have found with our clients that selecting one gift for all of the women and another for all of the men makes the task easier to comprehend. One of our clients felt very successful and fulfilled by sending each woman in his large family a scarf and each man a sweater. We were careful to buy the gifts at a major department store and slipped gift tags into the boxes so the recipients could exchange them as they wished. Our client could never recall what he had sent as gifts, but he benefited greatly from going through the process with his caregiver of selecting, purchasing, wrapping, and mailing each parcel to his widespread family.

Be a teammate

This is another opportunity to help your loved one avoid the withdrawal into passivity that results from recurrent failure. Selecting and preparing gifts is a process, one that includes multiple steps and provides repeated opportunities for experiencing success.

The goal is not to have all the presents wrapped and ready to mail or distribute on time. It is to see your loved one enjoy each step along the way—to have experienced the joy of selecting, wrapping, and sending gifts. If your loved one has experienced the endorphin rush that accompanies accomplishment, you have succeeded spectacularly—even if the parcels are late.

Focus on one step at a time

Dementia truly is the time for measuring success in terms of how enjoyable a task is rather than in its completion. When people are losing rational thought, they lose the ability to prioritize actions and information as well as the ability to follow directions and multiple steps in a sequence. Always focus on the single step at hand.

When we think of the holiday season as an experience to be enjoyed rather than as a series of tasks to be accomplished, we all discover moments of beauty along the way.

■ ■ ■

Music—Adding Comfort and Enjoyment to Dementia

Music reaches all of us emotionally. It can bring tears to our eyes, give us goose bumps, grate on our ears, calm us, or send us out of the room. People with dementia respond to music just as surely as people with healthy brains do. We do not need rational thought to respond to music.

However, rational thought is necessary to play a CD on the stereo or find your favorite music channel on the television. How can we help our loved ones who have dementia continue to access and enjoy the music that brings them enjoyment and comfort?

I am not very skilled at using technology. In my home, I still have a much-loved stereo and collection of CDs. At work, I have an original iPod loaded with my CD collection. Every day, I use my memory and thinking skills to operate my stereo and iPod. If you are with your loved one daily, you can use your skills to keep music in his or her life as well, but without your help, your loved one will become cut off from music.

Use the existing stereo or television

For clients in the earlier stages of dementia, we create CDs with a collection of their favorite pieces. For a time, they are able to put that one CD in the player. This ability soon goes, however. We also tune their televisions to their favorite music stations. Most cable services include music genre stations so you can select the ones your loved one enjoys.

Add an iPod Shuffle

The next step is to follow Dan Cohen's lead and turn to iTunes (see his work at musicandmemory.org) and the iPod Shuffle, a device that will play a random and continuous selection of whatever music it is programmed with. Since it has only an on/off button, someone with dementia can operate it successfully. We recommend that families purchase two Shuffles and load one with the music their loved one finds entertaining and the other with a selection of music that he or she finds calming and comforting.

Update the television with a streaming device

A world of music is accessible with a smart television or a streaming device. At present, the consensus is that streaming devices are the better investment.

I invested in a Roku device. The two channels I get the most enjoyment from are Pandora, a free music-streaming app, and YouTube, which can provide hours of long-running audio and video selections of music or nature. With Pandora, you create individual music channels and then train the channel to play only the music you prefer by clicking *like* or *dislike* with the remote. You can quickly and easily set up Pandora to provide an array of channels with music that will meet your loved one's every need.

YouTube also provides thousands of musical selections. More importantly, it provides a wealth of nature videos. You can stream hours of uninterrupted birdsong or the sounds of babbling brooks, forests, lakes, beaches—anything you can imagine from the natural world. When you let a selection play, you are prompting YouTube to offer you similar selections. I now have YouTube trained to offer crackling fires for chilly mornings, birdsong in meadows and gardens, sunsets over gentle waves, waterfalls, and forest walks—all with just a few clicks of the remote.

Adding a streaming device or smart television enables you to bring the beauty of music and nature into your loved one's home with a minimal initial investment and Internet access. The number of free music and nature streaming apps and websites is ever increasing.

■ ■ ■

On the Road with Dementia

Getting There in One Piece

Traveling can be stressful in the best of times. Taking someone who has dementia on a holiday or to visit family or friends can quickly become an ordeal. Whether you plan to drive to the next town or fly across the nation, take some time beforehand to think about how travel and change affect people who lack memory and rational thought.

When people lack rational thought, they are unable to perceive cause and effect, to follow a sequence, or to prioritize events or information. So, although it may be obvious to you that getting on an airplane and flying for several hours means that you will not be sleeping in your own bed that night, it is not likely that someone with dementia will see that as a certainty.

In addition, although for most of us there is at least a semblance of logic in the process of waiting at the ticket counter to check our bags, shuffling along in a security line, being frisked by a uniformed TSA agent, having our carry-ons gone through, and then waiting interminably at the gate for an overdue flight, such sequential events are not something people with dementia can understand and plod through easily. Frustration and meltdown are more likely to occur when something seems random and unfathomable.

Further, deadlines mean nothing when you cannot track time or read clocks; meeting them is even less likely when you cannot see that putting shoes on is essential but drinking a cup of coffee is not. All of this means that when we take a loved one with dementia away from what is familiar and routine, we will need to keep up a cheerful monologue about what is happening—and what can be expected next—all along the way. When we do this, we are using our own rational thought skills to make up for what our loved ones have lost. This ready stream of information helps our loved ones continue to feel comfortable despite lacking memory and the skills that rational thought provides.

"Where are we?"

Without memory, we live entirely in the present. So, if we find ourselves in unfamiliar surroundings, our natural reaction is concern—or at least curiosity—and we will have that reaction every time we realize that we do not know where we are. The psychological present is about three seconds. Although a small child might be bored and ask several times how much longer the trip will last, someone experiencing dementia is likely to feel fearful in unfamiliar surroundings and need constant reassurance for the duration of the time spent away from home.

"Do you need to use the bathroom?"

When someone is experiencing dementia, he or she may not be able to interpret feelings such as hunger or the urge to use the bathroom. So, although we may be able to trust a child's report of not needing to go, people with dementia might say no and truly not realize that they do need a bathroom until after an accident occurs. Our approach is to say that we need to use the bathroom ourselves; often, once we are there, our clients realize they would like to as well. However, it is always wise to carry wipes and a change of clothes for possible emergencies.

Getting lost in a restaurant

Even people in the earlier stages of dementia can become flustered and lost when they walk out of a bathroom in a restaurant or any strange place. Be sure to keep an eye out to see that your loved one finds the way back to your table or back to her bedroom in a strange home. In the panic of not knowing which way to turn upon leaving the bathroom, she may become unable to recognize familiar faces as well and head for an exit.

Should we leave home at all?

You may now be wondering whether you want to travel with someone who has dementia. It requires careful planning as well as keeping a close watch on your loved one's reactions as he or she meets so much new information and stimuli. However, if you make sure that someone is always on duty—watching for ways to ensure that security needs and understanding needs are met—travel can be enjoyable. Try to have more than just one person available for caregiving. In addition, recognize that stress and change exacerbate memory loss and confusion, so your loved one will function less well when away from the familiarities of home.

■ ■ ■

Turning No into Yes

Reaching Underlying Issues of Disempowerment

People do not like being told what to do. That does not change when dementia appears. When someone demands that we do something, our initial response is an inward, momentary "Why should I?" or "Who are you to tell me what to do?" Dementia does not take away those innate feelings of personal autonomy. It only takes away the reasoning and acceptance that follows that initial response when we have rational thought skills.

Worse, dementia can affect the part of the brain that gives us self-awareness, so people experiencing dementia are often unaware of their impairments. When people are unaware that they lack memory or good judgment, they are even more resistant to taking direction from others, even though it is often to their detriment.

What can we do to help our loved ones and clients willingly choose to do the things we know are in their best interests?

Create independence

There are ways to enhance someone's feelings of empowerment. When dementia takes away memory and rational thought functions, it becomes difficult to make decisions. If we ask our loved ones or clients open-ended questions, we are compounding their difficulties. Open-ended questions, such as "What do you want for lunch," require the use of recall and analysis to come up with an answer.

It is much easier for someone with dementia to choose between two options or to choose whether to do something or not. So, a kind caregiver will ask, "Would you like a cookie or piece of pie?" rather than asking, "What to do you want for dessert?" And, "Would you like to go for a walk?" rather than, "What would you like to do?" Asking open-ended questions inhibits the ability to exercise choice; presenting options enables it. In essence, the caregiver is using his or her own rational thought and memory skills on behalf of the loved one or client. Using questions to present options and choices is a way we can empower someone with dementia.

Make options visible

Another empowering technique that caregivers can use is to be thoughtful about what is visible and what is not visible in the home. Clutter or too many visual options in the kitchen, bedroom, or bathroom inhibit the ability to choose. Clear off surfaces and put out just the items you want used or selected. Lay out a favorite or appropriate outfit on the bed. Put away everything by the sink except the toothbrush and toothpaste. Set a place at the table with a sandwich and finger food visible under plastic wrap; pour the glass of milk or cup of coffee.

Making options visible removes the need for recall, selection, and deliberation. It provides more opportunities to exercise choice.

Don't mention the end goal

Does your loved one or client routinely refuse to shower or dress or attend medical appointments? Several emotional needs can cause refusals, but when an activity is consistently refused, we need to reconsider our approach.

One of our clients does not like going down the hall to the bathroom, most likely because she's susceptible to urinary tract infections and often has pain on voiding. She associates pain with using the toilet. So, her caregiver never asks her directly. Rather, she suggests that they go look in the mirror so she can fix her hair. Our client loves having her hair done and will often use the toilet without complaint once she is in the bathroom.

When we feel out of control, our need to regain control, even in small ways, increases. Conversely, when we are routinely presented with options and given the ability to choose, we feel less need for control overall. Good dementia care means proactively thinking about ways to increase our clients' sense of control. We will experience less stress, as well.

■ ■ ■

My purpose in developing the DAWN Method and making it available was to give families and caregivers awareness and understanding of the emotional needs caused by dementia, and the ability to put habilitative care into practice at home. I want to equip all of us with the tools and techniques that will help people with dementia preserve autonomy, dignity, and personal safety. I want to enable all of us to stay in our own homes for longer.

Habilitative care, with its acceptance of both the skills that remain and those lost in dementia, is not only the most economical and kindest but also the most commonsense way to care for people who have dementia.

CHAPTER 5
Why Should We?

I hope I have now given you a glimpse of how easily we can live with people who are experiencing dementia and improve not only their quality of life but ours as caregivers as well. The question I hope I've answered is why it is so important that we learn how to care for our loved ones ourselves and keep them home for as long as we can. In summary, here are the three primary reasons we should.

We Can't Afford Long-Term Care

Let's consider the cost of long-term care in terms of earning potential. As an attorney practicing elder law in Portland, Oregon, in the late 2000s, I settled quite a few estates. I didn't have an upper-crust clientele. The families who came to me knew they needed an attorney to see that the deceased's assets and liabilities were properly disposed of. They also hoped to see the estate settled out of the proceeds.

I think back on those families as representative of middle-class Americans for their generation. Typically, the deceased would be a father who had worked in one occupation or for one or two companies his entire adult life, or a mother who was a stay-at-home mom and might have gone to work after the children were grown. The deceased had usually been living in the family home, which was paid for, and had retirement accounts and savings in about the $300,000 range.

There were two scenarios. In the first, long-term care had not been needed and the estate would be settled with some inheritance for the next generation. In the second, one of the parents had developed dementia or needed long-term care for a medical reason. At an average cost of $90,500 per year, this family had seen its assets consumed by the cost of long-term care. The children would receive no inheritance and would pay the cost of estate settlement out of their own pockets.

Yet in both situations, the children probating their parents' estates needed an inheritance much more than their parents did. A study conducted at Stanford University in 2016 showed that we baby boomers are not as well off as our parents. People born in the 1940s could expect to earn more than their parents—to live the American dream—but subsequent generations have had less success. The generation I probated estates for could have chosen to attend college at little expense, pay off a mortgage during their working years, and save for retirement. They could plan to live on those savings and their social-security income when they retired. However, only about 75 percent of those born in the 1950s achieved as much earning power as their parents. For those born in the 1980s and later, only about half make as much money as their parents.

We simply are not able to afford to institutionalize people who develop dementia at the rate that we have been, because fewer of us have the economic means. Worse yet, dementia is an epidemic, so more and more families are finding themselves in the second situation above. Economics are forcing us to care for our loved ones at home. We have no choice but to equip ourselves to provide more effective dementia care.

However, as I hope I've demonstrated, providing effective dementia care isn't beyond our reach. We can do it at home or bring in caregivers to help our loved ones stay in their own homes. Effective dementia care comes from recognizing and accepting the parameters dementia creates—the cognitive abilities that remain and the ones that fade away. When we provide care that supports both, stress is minimized for both caregivers and care receivers, and it becomes possible to postpone institutional care.

Person-Directed Care Is Kinder

The role of providing care is to recognize a person's needs and meet them. When we, here in America, began using the appropriate-care approach and reality orientation with people experiencing dementia, we didn't intend to be unkind. Reality orientation works quite well with people who have mental illnesses or have experienced traumatic brain injuries. We use it on ourselves when we awake from a deep sleep or vivid dream. It is time to accept, however, that it does not work with people who have lost rational thought.

Without rational thought, our loved ones who have dementia are not equipped to respond to reality orientation. It's no different than expecting a toddler to sit quietly for an opera, a college student to turn his social calendar over to his parents, or someone recovering from a hip replacement to enjoy an afternoon spent ice skating in the park. In each situation, we are asking someone to do what they cannot do—either physically or psychologically—which is a profound unkindness. The kinder and more sensible response is to take into account each person's limitations and change the environment to meet the individual's needs. That is the essence of habilitative care.

We need to remind ourselves that, just like the examples above, dementia is not a disease. Although it may result from a disease, it is something that cannot be cured at present. Dementia is a condition, one that does not cause us to need medical care until the latest stages. It does, however, very quickly put us in need of companions who can recognize and support our changing abilities and disabilities.

When we persist in viewing dementia as something best dealt with by doctors and nurses, we sacrifice quality of life for extension of life. However, a life devoid of the things that fulfill us and give us a sense of well-being is psychologically painful. We need autonomy and dignity, beauty and sensory stimulation, and contact with others through meaningful relationships and physical touch. It is much easier to keep what is important to us within reach when we live in our own homes and communities; yet, when I meet with families to design care plans, usually someone will eventually say, "She should be in a nursing home." I always ask why. Invariably the first answer is that it would be safer. When I point out that statistically care facilities are not safer than private homes, the answer becomes, "She's too old to live at home."

Why do we think that? Children are also unable to care for themselves properly, but we don't believe they would be safer living in boarding schools. Many of our clients have continued to live in their own homes, some through death, yet we have very little experience with sundowning or wandering. Not one has died of neglect, abuse, or due to an accident. When we design care to meet our clients' sensory and social stimulation needs, they reach the end of the day feeling content and fulfilled. They experience both safety and quality of life, because we have succeeded in supporting both their abilities and disabilities.

When people develop dementia, they need their families and caregivers to provide them with habilitative care. Only those who know them can truly design or provide the kind of care that supports who they are, helps them continue to experience what brings them quality of life, and preserves their autonomy. Institutional care should be the last resort, when all other options have been exhausted.

It's Time to Honor Elderhood

We live in a society that prizes rational thought over intuitive thought and accomplishment over experiences and relationships. We accept childhood as the time for developing the skills we need to become successful adults and see adulthood as the time for being productive and accumulating assets. We don't think about elderhood very much, but, when we do, we think about those experiencing it as people who are failing at adulthood rather than succeeding at elderhood.

Yet elderhood is as valuable a part of life as childhood and adulthood. It is the time for being rather than doing, for reflection rather than accomplishment, for sharing rather than accumulating. Our elders have a lifetime of experience and learning to share with us. When dementia comes into the picture, they need respectful support. I fear, however, that before we can revise our concept of dementia care to encompass identifying and meeting the specific needs that arise with dementia, we must first begin seeing elderhood as a life stage worthy of our respect. We're predisposed to not appreciate elderhood due to our focus on productivity, and we ignore the valuable skills dementia leaves untouched due to our admiration of rational thought.

Maybe our society has little appreciation for the final stage in life because we tend to segregate generations. Not many of us grew up in a three-generation home. We send our children off to daycare and preschool, sometimes from infancy, where they are socialized by their peers rather than grandparents. The one-room schoolhouse is a thing of the past. Yet each generation brings enrichment to the others. My closest friends range from twenty-two to eighty-eight, and my life is enriched by each one of them.

When I am with my clients, I am amazed by their capacity to enjoy beauty in all its forms, even if they were not very aware of it earlier in life. I find spending time with them uplifting because I join them in savoring what we encounter in the present. We might need to buy groceries or get to a medical appointment, but we notice how blue the sky is along the way. I come to them with joy and anticipation, and they join me wholeheartedly. I am frequently struck, however, by how seldom family members see their loved ones' newfound sensitivity to beauty or the effect that their own sadness and frustration has on their loved ones' moods.

My life has been enriched immeasurably by my clients. They have taught me so much—from courage in the absence of hope to a fail-proof way to get coffee stains out of a white shirt, from resilience in the face of constant failure to how to grow juicier tomatoes in northern Idaho. Being without rational thought has never prevented my clients from being fully human. In their moments of clarity, we share profound truths. The rest of the time, I use my rational thought and memory to help them continue to function with intuitive thought alone. At the beginning of this book, I said that over the past six years I have spent more time with people who have dementia than with people who don't have it. I am so glad I did. It was never a burden. I have been enriched, educated, and guided by my clients—not in spite of their dementia but because of it.

Dementia is bad, but not all bad. There is still much to be shared if we understand that our loved ones are not losing their intuitive thought skills or their experiential selves. We can continue to live with them and care for them when we focus on the skills they retain rather than on those they are losing. There is hope in dementia. It lies in the way we provide care.

GLOSSARY

Alzheimer's disease:
Alzheimer's is one of the diseases that cause dementia. It results primarily in problems with memory and, like all forms of dementia, in problems with thinking and behavior. Symptoms usually develop slowly and get worse over time, becoming severe enough to interfere with daily tasks. Alzheimer's disease is the most common cause of dementia in the United States.

Anosognosia:
The condition of being unable to perceive or be aware of one's physical or neurological deficits. In dementia, people are often aware that they have memory problems but are unable to comprehend that they have problems with using judgment or rational thought.

Appropriate care:
A term used in the United States to identify health care in which the expected clinical benefits outweigh the expected negative effects, justifying the treatment. This has been the default approach in dementia care and senior care facilities. The hallmark of the appropriate-care approach is reality orientation, which asks people with dementia to accept our common reality although they do not have the necessary cognitive skills (memory and rational thought) to perceive it.

Automatic thinking scripts:
The ability to mindlessly complete a routine task without thinking about the individual steps. Automatic thinking scripts are created by repetition. People experiencing dementia continue to be able to

perform routine tasks using automatic thinking scripts, as long as there is no interruption or change to the setting.

Dementia:

Dementia is a condition, not a disease. It is a descriptive term for a collection of symptoms that can be caused by a number of disorders that affect the brain. People with dementia have significantly impaired intellectual functioning (loss of rational thought) that interferes with normal activities and relationships. They lose their ability to solve problems and maintain emotional control, and they may experience personality changes and behavioral problems. Memory loss by itself does not mean that a person has dementia. Doctors diagnose dementia only if two or more brain functions, such as memory and language skills, are significantly impaired.

Experiential self:

The part of us that is in the present, experiencing what is occurring to us and around us. The experiential self is absorbing information from the five physical senses even if we are not able to make sense of the stimuli we are receiving, describe what we are experiencing, or express what we are feeling.

Fight-or-flight response:

The fight-or-flight response, also known as the acute stress response, is a physiological reaction that occurs in the presence of something that is terrifying, either mentally or physically. The response is triggered by the release of hormones that prepare your body to either stay and deal with a threat or run away to safety.

Habilitative care:
The opposite of the appropriate-care approach. We are using habilitative care when we accept people's abilities and disabilities and change the environment to make it safer and more comfortable for them. Caregivers who are habilitative in their approach focus on their charges' individual interpretations of reality rather than requiring acceptance of our common reality. They focus on meeting their charges' emotional needs and preserving dignity and autonomy.

Intuitive thought processes:
Intuitive thought processes are our System 1 thought processes, sometimes referred to as our right brain. Intuitive thought operates automatically, instantaneously, and without effort. It is the source of our feelings, impressions, and gut reactions. We are using our intuitive thought skills when we read intonation, facial expressions, and body language. Intuitive thought is our means of enjoying music and beauty. It includes our ability to learn by experience.

Mindfulness:
According to Ellen Langer, "Mindfulness is a flexible state of mind in which we are actively engaged in the present, noticing new things." It comes from being able to use rational thought to focus or pay attention.

Mindlessness:
When we are not actively engaged in what we are doing, we are acting unconsciously and following a series of steps or behaving without conscious decision.

Muscle memory:

The ability to mindlessly follow a route or the steps in a task that we have performed many times before. Our muscles are following the pattern without conscious direction. When we ask someone to pay attention, muscle memory is interrupted and lost.

Person-directed care:

Dementia care that is based on a person's specific and changing personal needs rather than dictated by schedules, protocols, or norms. The person-directed caregiver supports the care receiver's abilities and provides targeted assistance in the areas where help is needed. This not only meets the person's needs but also supports his or her interests.

Rational thought processes:

Our System 2 thought processes, sometimes referred to as our left brain. Rational thought is our conscious, reasoning self. With it we can analyze data, be methodical, make choices, see cause and effect, prioritize information and actions, and follow a process or series of steps. Rational thought is not instantaneous; it takes effort. Rational thought will also tell us whether our behavior is appropriate for the circumstance and includes our ability to learn by rote.

Reality Orientation:

The act of correcting a person's mistaken beliefs about reality by telling them when they are mistaken about where they are, what time or day it is, what has happened, is happening or about to happen. It was used first with severely disturbed war veterans and continues to be used with people with traumatic brain injuries, mental illnesses, and dementia in the United States. Although it is effective when used with people who retain the ability to use memory skills and rational thought skills, it is usually met with resistance when people lack the rational thought skills necessary to accept an explanation of reality that differs from what their own brains are telling them.

Remembering self:
The part of us that enjoys looking back and recalling earlier times. It is nostalgic and provides us with the sense of familiarity in our surroundings. Our remembering selves shape our view of the present by providing verification and explanations drawn from our past experiences.

DEMENTIA FLOWCHART

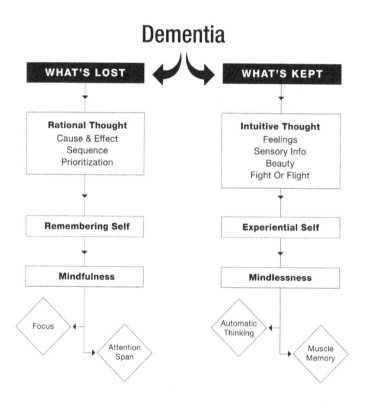

DEMENTIA OUTLINE

1. What is lost:
   a. Memory and recall:
      i. Memories that disappear.
      ii. Memories that become changed.
   b. Remembering self:
      i. Knowledge of the past.
   c. Rational thought processes:
      i. Cause and effect.
      ii. Sequence or steps in series.
      iii. Prioritization of action and ideas.
   d. Language skills:
      i. Word choice.
      ii. Vocabulary.
      iii. Comprehension of others' speech.
   e. Motor skills:
      i. Dexterity.
      ii. Coordination.

2. What isn't lost:
   a. Intuitive thought processes:
      i. Feeling and responding to emotions and moods:
         1. Feeling one's own feelings and moods.
         2. Reading feelings and moods of others.
      ii. Enjoying beauty.
      iii. Receiving sensory feedback.
      iv. Fight-or-flight response.

b. Experiential self:

    i. Psychological present (three seconds).

c. Mindlessness:

    i. Automatic thinking scripts.

    ii. Muscle memory.

DAWN DEMENTIA CARE

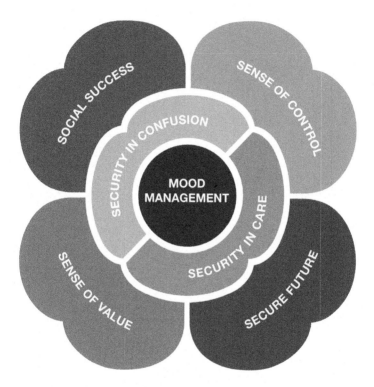

See the DAWN Method in use at www.thedawnmethod.com.

BIBLIOGRAPHY

Gawande, Atul. *Being Mortal.* London: Profile Books, 2014.

Kahneman, Daniel. *Thinking, Fast and Slow.* New York: Farrar, Straus and Giroux, 2011.

Koenig Coste, Joanne. *Learning to Speak Alzheimer's.* New York: Houghton Mifflin Harcourt, 2003.

Langer, Ellen. *Mindfulness.* Philadelphia: Da Capo Press, 2014.

Power, Allen. *Dementia beyond Drugs.* Baltimore, MD: Health Professions Press, 2014.

Shaughnessy, Mina. *Errors and Expectations.* New York: Oxford University Press, 1977.

Tolle, Eckhart. *The Power of Now.* Vancouver: Namaste Publishing, 1999.

Cohen, Dan. "Our Mission and Vision." Music & Memory, Inc. www.musicandmemory.org (accessed January 23, 2017).

Made in the USA
Las Vegas, NV
19 May 2023